ABDOMINAL INCISIONS AND THEIR CLOSURE

HAROLD ELLIS, D.M., M.Ch., F.R.C.S.
TIMOTHY E. BUCKNALL, M.S., F.R.C.S.
PETER J. COX, B.Sc., F.R.C.S.

0011-3840/85/04-001-051-$9.95
© 1985, Year Book Medical Publishers, Inc.

CONTENTS

FOREWORD. 3

SELF-ASSESSMENT QUESTIONS 4

CLASSIFICATION OF ABDOMINAL INCISIONS. 6

OPERATIVE TECHNIQUES OF ABDOMINAL INCISIONS 8

DISRUPTION OF THE ABDOMINAL WALL 17

TECHNICAL FACTORS IN BURST ABDOMEN 22

MORTALITY FROM BURST ABDOMEN 27

INCISIONAL HERNIA. 28

CHOICE OF SUTURE MATERIAL 30

TECHNIQUES OF CLOSURE 43

SELF-ASSESSMENT ANSWERS. 51

FOREWORD

The abdominal incision is often described in excessive detail by the novice surgeon and hardly mentioned by the expert surgeon in their respective operative notes—a simple fact that best demonstrates the various preoccupations and levels of expertise at the beginning of an operation. The authors put the importance of a well placed and carefully executed incision into the right perspective, show the advantages and disadvantages of various incisions in the conduct of the operative procedure itself, and demonstrate that a reliable and safe closure is based on many factors, including the care with which the incision was traced at the very beginning of the operation. Their studies in comparing various wound closure techniques and materials should eliminate many inherited and acquired myths; they have already done so for the present reviewer who nevertheless is bemoaning the fate of the gentle, soft, pliable silk thread.

FELICIEN M. STEICHEN, M.D.
ASSOCIATE EDITOR

SELF-ASSESSMENT QUESTIONS

1. Which of the following sutures are absorbable?
   a. Polydioxanone.
   b. Polypropylene.
   c. Polyglactin.
2. Significant factors associated with wound failure include:
   a. Infection.
   b. Obesity.
   c. Uremia.
3. The frequency of sinus formation is directly related to the degree of contamination. True or false?
4. Abdominal wall fascia heals in:
   a. 14 days.
   b. 30 days.
   c. 120 days.
5. The commonest cause of suture failure is:
   a. Material failure.
   b. Iatrogenic, due to rough handling.
   c. Tissue effect on suture.
6. Pfannenstiel is German for "bucket handle." True or false?
7. The lateral paramedian incision can be employed for all abdominal surgery. True or false?
8. Which of the following incisions have an unacceptably high incisional hernia rate?
   a. Gridiron (McBurney).
   b. Midline.
   c. Full-length wide paramedian.
   d. Transverse.
   e. Conventional paramedian.
9. Chromic catgut retains more than 50% of its strength in vivo for:
   a. 7 days.
   b. 14 days.
   c. 28 days.
10. In mass closure:
   a. The bites should be at least 1 cm deep.
   b. The bites should be at least ½ cm deep.
   c. The length of suture used should be less than four times the wound length.

Answers appear at the end of the article.

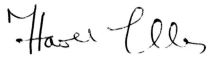

is Professor of Surgery at the University of London. He is the Chairman of the Department of Surgery of Charing Cross and Westminster Medical School in London. Dr. Ellis is also civilian Consultant Surgeon to the Army and Member of Council, Royal College of Surgeons of England.

Timothy Annan

is a senior surgical registrar at Westminster Hospital in London, England.

Peter J Cose

is a senior surgical registrar at Westminster Hospital in London, England.

ESTABLISHING efficient access to the abdominal cavity and the safe closure of the consequent wound are two vital, if somewhat neglected, steps in the performance of every laparotomy. Unfortunately, the approach to the abdominal cavity is often selected without much thought, and closure of the wound, especially at the end of a long and testing operation, may be carried out with less than meticulous care.

A well-planned incision allows (1) excellent access to the planned field of operation, (2) the possibility of extension of the exposure if some unforeseen problem arises, and (3) safe closure to be performed.

In turn, effective closure should be a relatively simple and speedy technique but one that is compatible with a low risk of incisional hernia, hematoma, infection, or, most serious of all, complete disruption of the laparotomy wound. In addition, the technique should provide a comfortable and reasonably aesthetic scar.

Ideally, closure of the incision should leave the abdominal wall as strong after operation as before, and this depends not only on the technique of closure but also on the choice of suture material and on careful planning in the placement of drains or stomas, should either of these be necessary.

In this monograph, we consider first the various approaches to the abdominal cavity, their description, and their advantages and disadvantages, then the problems of abdominal closure (burst abdomen, incisional hernia, sinuses), and finally the choice of suture materials and techniques of closure. Wherever possible the results of various methods are presented on the basis of controlled trials, carried out by ourselves and by other surgical investigators, rather than on that most dangerous barrier to scientific progress, the "clinical impression."

CLASSIFICATION OF ABDOMINAL INCISIONS

The common incisions used in exploring the abdominal cavity may be grouped into vertical incisions and transverse and oblique incisions. Vertical incisions may be of the midline (median), paramedian (either rectus sliding or rectus splitting), or wide paramedian type. These incisions may be supraumbilical or infraumbilical or may extend the full length of the abdominal cavity. Transverse and oblique incisions include McBurney's muscle-splitting incision, Kocher's subcostal incision (right or left), other oblique (Rutherford-Morrison) or transverse muscle-cutting incisions, and the Pfannenstiel infraumbilical incision. Both the vertical upper abdominal and the oblique upper abdominal incisions can be extended through the right or left chest to fashion thoracoabdominal incisions.

CHOICE OF INCISION

Many factors must be taken into consideration in planning the laparotomy incision. How certain is the surgeon of the diagnosis and of the procedure to be carried out? Is speed a vital consideration in some life-threatening emergency? What is the build of the patient (particularly, what is the subcostal angle, and what is the degree of obesity)? Are there previous abdominal incisions? Will an abdominal stoma be required? No rigid rules can be laid down, and in many cases the choice of the incision depends on the surgeon's preference.

Provided that the preoperative diagnosis is confirmed, there is no doubt that the McBurney right iliac fossa muscle-splitting incision is ideal for appendectomy. It is easy to create, gives good access, can be closed speedily and with ease, leaves a hairline skin crease scar, virtually never disrupts, and is rarely the site of an incisional hernia, unless a large drain has been brought out directly through the wound. If necessary the incision can be readily enlarged, either medially or laterally.

Similarly, the Pfannenstiel incision is excellent for local gynecologic conditions, but the exposure is undoubtedly limited and the incision should not be employed when a maneuver outside the pelvis may be required.

The Kocher subcostal incision provides excellent access to the gallbladder and biliary duct system in obese patients with a wide subcostal angle. However, in the thin patient with a narrow subcostal angle, there is little advantage over a vertical incision. Similarly, the paramedian incision does provide better access than the midline incision for treating pathologic conditions in the right and left flanks in obese and muscular patients, whereas the paramedian incision offers little advantage over the midline approach in thin subjects.

The midline vertical incision is the one most commonly employed throughout the surgical world. It is easy to create and easy to close, almost bloodless, quick, provides exposure to every abdominal and retroperitoneal viscus, and can if necessary be extended from the xiphoid to the pubis by skirting around the umbilicus.[1] However, the midline incision is often denigrated as being the one that carries the highest risk of burst abdomen and incisional hernia formation, and for this reason the other approaches we have listed are thought by some to be less susceptible to these complications. These virtues are brought forward in counterargument to the undoubted fact that they are more tedious to create and to close than the midline incision.

In earlier published accounts of wound dehiscence, the midline incision figures prominently in the statistics. However, the reason may not be too hard to find: these studies, being uncontrolled, made no allowance for the fact that often the midline incision is carried out in cases of the greatest urgency—hemorrhage, trauma, sepsis—or in reopening previous laparotomy wounds, perhaps already the site of an incisional hernia. The other, more sophisticated incisions tend to be employed in selected and elective cases. Therefore, we can hardly be surprised that more complications have been found in the former than in the latter group.

As we shall later discuss, prospective controlled clinical trials have shown that, in respect to wound dehiscence or hernia formation, there is little or nothing to choose between the results obtained from midline, paramedian, and oblique or transverse incisions. The only approach having an undoubted advantage in this respect is the recently introduced wide or lateral paramedian incision.[2]

Re-entry into the abdominal cavity should, whenever possible, be performed through the previous incision, especially if this is already weak or the site of an incisional hernia, since re-entry here enables repair to be carried out at the same time. There is a definite risk that a second incision placed beside the previous wound, especially if heavily undercut, may compromise the blood supply of the skin between the two incisions, leading to necrosis of the intervening skin bridge.

OPERATIVE TECHNIQUES OF ABDOMINAL INCISIONS

The Muscle-Splitting Incision

The muscle-splitting incision is the incision of choice in most cases of acute appendicitis. It was described by McBurney in 1894.[3] It gives excellent access, is easily extended and readily closed, and is followed by good healing and cosmesis and virtually no risk of subsequent wound disruption or herniation.

Classically, the incision is centered at McBurney's point (Fig 1), which is the junction of the middle and outer one-third of the line running from the umbilicus to the anterior superior iliac spine. However, if palpation of the abdomen under anesthesia reveals a mass, the incision should be placed directly over the mass. The length of the incision will vary according to the obesity of the patient, and may therefore range from 3 to 12 cm or more. Originally the skin incision was placed obliquely from above and laterally to below medially, and indeed this placement is still used if the patient is obese or if it is anticipated that lateral extension of the incision may be necessary as a muscle-cutting incision. Usually, however, the incision is placed transversely in the line of the skin crease, which gives a better cosmetic result.

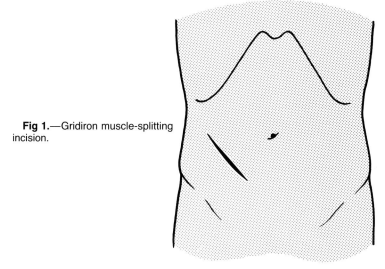

Fig 1.—Gridiron muscle-splitting incision.

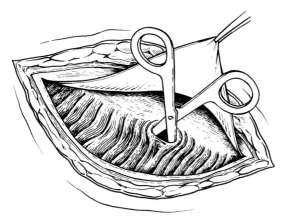

Fig 2.—Muscle-splitting incision. External oblique muscle has been split in the direction of its fibers. A small incision is made and the underlying fibers are split using scissors or artery forceps (clamp).

Skin and subcutaneous fat are divided, then the external oblique aponeurosis is split in the direction of its fibers. A small incision is then made immediately adjacent to the outer border of the rectus sheath and the internal oblique and transversus fibers are split open in the line of their fibers, using scissors or artery forceps (hemostatic clamp) (Fig 2), revealing the underlying peritoneum. The intact peritoneum is separated from the transversus muscle by blunt fingertip dissection, gently elevating the edges of the muscle. This maneuver relaxes the peritoneum and facilitates incision as well as closure of the peritoneum, which is now picked up between artery forceps (clamps) and opened with the scalpel. The opening is enlarged by means of the two index fingers (Fig 3), which produces a circular hole in the peritoneum that can be readily closed with a purse string or running suture at the end of the operation.

Further access is easily obtained medially by dividing the anterior rectus sheath in line with the incision, after which the rectus muscle can be retracted medially. Wide lateral extension of the incision can be effected by a combination of division and splitting of the oblique muscles along the line of their fibers. On the left side, this extended muscle-splitting incision is particularly suitable as an approach to lesions of the sigmoid colon.

THE MIDLINE INCISION

Virtually any operation in the abdominal cavity can be performed through this universally applicable incision, which has the advantages of being almost bloodless and quick to create and close (so that it is of immense value in cases of great urgency). The incision can be extended the full length of the abdomen if it

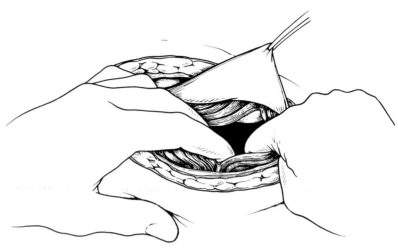

Fig 3.—Muscle-splitting incision. The opening is enlarged by means of the two index fingers.

is curved around the umbilicus, and it is made without division of either muscle fibers or nerves.

In the upper abdomen, the incision is placed exactly in the midline and extends downward from the xiphisternum, usually to end immediately above the umbilicus. Skin, fat, linea alba, extraperitoneal fat, and peritoneum are divided. Division of the peritoneum is best carried out at the lower extremity of the wound so that the falciform ligament can be seen and avoided. If this ligament interferes with exposure, it should be divided between clamps and ligated. Upward extension of a few centimeters can be achieved by running the incision to one or other side of the xiphoid process.

The subumbilical incision differs only in that here the linea alba is usually very narrow, so that the rectus sheath on one or the other side may be inadvertently opened, although this is not of any consequence. In the lower abdomen the peritoneum should be opened first in its upper part to avoid possible injury to the bladder.

Special care must be taken in opening the peritoneum under two circumstances—and this applies to all laparotomy incisions, not only the midline incision. First, in cases of intestinal obstruction, loops of distended bowel immediately deep to the peritoneum may be injured and the initial opening into the peritoneal cavity must be made with the greatest care. Second, great care is required when the abdomen is reopened following a previous operation. In the majority of cases, there will be underlying adhesions, and if these include intestine, the gut may inadvertently be injured. The peritoneum should be opened at one or the other end of the incision, away from the immediate mass of adhesions. Once the peritoneal cavity has been safely entered, the peritoneal edges are held up with artery forceps and the adhesions are detached under direct vision.

THE CONVENTIONAL PARAMEDIAN INCISION

The upper paramedian incision, on either the right or the left side, usually commences at the costal margin and is taken down to the level of the umbilicus, or lower. It is placed 1–2 inches (2.5–5 cm) from the midline. Additional access can be obtained by sloping the incision upward and inward as far as the xiphoid (Fig 4).

Skin and subcutaneous fat are divided along the length of the wound. The anterior rectus sheath is exposed and incised and its medial edge is grasped and lifted up by several artery forceps (clamps). The inner portion of the rectus sheath is now dissected from the rectus muscle, to which the anterior sheath adheres. Blood vessels are encountered at the three fibrous intersections of the rectus, placed just below the xiphoid, at the level of the umbilicus and halfway between. These vessels should be picked up and coagulated or ligated before they are divided. Once the rectus is free of the anterior sheath the muscle can be drawn laterally, since the posterior rectus sheath is not adherent to the back of the rectus muscle. The posterior sheath and peritoneum, which are intimately adherent to each other, are picked up and incised vertically for the whole length of the incision, deep to the medial longitudinal axis of the rectus muscle, to cover the peritoneal closure later. (the peritoneal closure may also be covered with muscle.)

The lower paramedian incision is very similar and, in fact, can

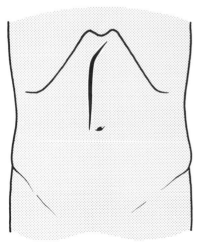

Fig 4.—Conventional paramedian incision. Extra access can be obtained by sloping the incision upward and inward as far as the xiphoid.

continue the upper paramedian incision the whole length of the abdomen. The only slight difference is that the inferior epigastric vessels are exposed in the posterior compartment of the rectus sheath and require ligation and division. Moreover, the posterior layer of the rectus sheath is deficient below the semilunar fold of Douglas in the lower half of the incision.

Some surgeons prefer to split the rectus muscle rather than dissecting it free and displacing it laterally. In this technique, the muscle is split longitudinally near its medial border and the peritoneum is opened in the same line. The advantage is that the incision can be quickly made and closed, an advantage shared with the technically simpler and more versatile midline incision. However, the rectus muscle-splitting incision is particularly useful in reopening the scar of a previous paramedian incision, when it is often very difficult or impossible to dissect the rectus muscle away from the scar tissue of the sheath and only a muscle-splitting incision is possible under these conditions.

There is the objection that such an incision may weaken the rectus muscle by separating the narrow medial strip of muscle from its lateral vascular and nerve supply. We have failed to find any controlled trial comparing the results of this rectus split incision with the conventional paramedian muscle slide procedure.

The Lateral Paramedian Incision

Recently, Guillou and his colleagues of St. James Hospital, Leeds, England, have described an interesting and important modification of the standard paramedian incision.[2] The vertical incision is placed at the junction of the middle and outer thirds of the width of the rectus sheath (Figs 5 and 6). The anterior sheath is incised and, in this situation, is found to consist of two layers. It is dissected from the rectus muscle (Fig 7), which is slid laterally in the usual fashion. The posterior sheath and peritoneum are divided in the same plane as the anterior sheath. The advantage the authors claim for such a laterally placed incision is that a very wide shutter mechanism is provided by the rectus muscle which should diminish the risk of burst abdomen and incisional hernia.

This is not an easy incision to perform and it certainly takes longer both to carry out and to close than other conventional incisions. Access is rather more restricted unless the incision is made quite long and, if necessary, angled medially toward the xiphoid in the upper abdomen or toward the pubis in a lower lateral paramedian incision. The value of the incision stands or falls on its ability to reduce dehiscence and incisional hernia formation. Our own controlled trials, described below, evidently

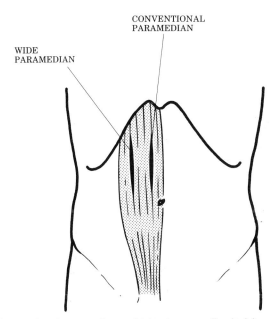

Fig 5.—Conventional paramedian and lateral paramedian incisions compared.

are the only ones that have been carried out outside of Leeds comparing this incision with conventional approaches, and our preliminary results support the excellent results claimed by the Leeds group.

THE SUBCOSTAL INCISION

The subcostal incision was described by Theodor Kocher of Berne, Switzerland.[4] It gives excellent exposure on the right side to the gallbladder and biliary tract and on the left side to the spleen. It is of special value in obese and muscular subjects.

The incision commences at the midline 1–2 inches (2.5–5 cm) below the xiphisternum and is continued downward and out-

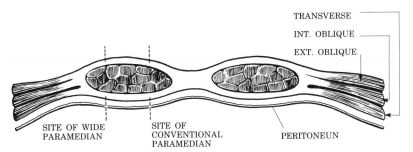

Fig 6.—Conventional paramedian and lateral paramedian incisions compared.

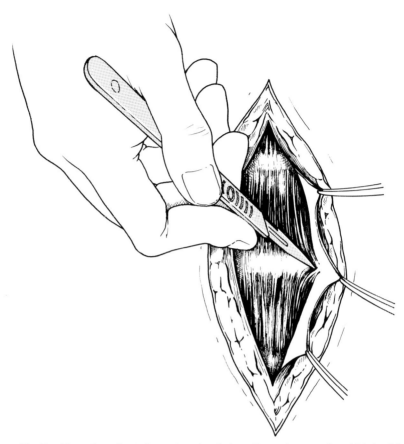

Fig 7.—Dissection of anterior rectus sheath from the rectus muscle, which is slid laterally in the usual fashion.

ward parallel and about 1 inch (2.5 cm) below the costal margin (Fig 8). The rectus sheath is incised and the rectus is divided the length of the incision, with diathermy coagulation used to control the branches of the superior epigastric vessels. The oblique abdominal muscles are divided in an outward direction for a short distance (Fig 9). The small eighth thoracic nerve is divided, but the large ninth nerve must be seen and preserved in order to prevent weakness of the abdominal musculature. The incision is then deepened and the peritoneum opened.

If necessary, the incision may be continued across the midline as an inverted V. This provides excellent access to the upper abdomen, for example in performing total abdominal gastrectomy in a particularly obese patient or in giving access to both suprarenal glands. However, with this incision both eighth thoracic nerves are divided and the potential of injury to the ninth nerve and subsequent muscle weakness is doubled.

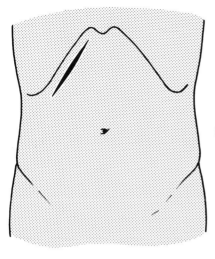

Fig 8.—Kocher's subcostal incision.

TRANSVERSE AND OBLIQUE MUSCLE-CUTTING INCISIONS

A transverse muscle-cutting incision can be used satisfactorily to expose intra-abdominal structures by dividing all the tissues in the line of the transverse skin incision. The incision must be long enough to give the required exposure.

For limited exposure in planned procedures a transverse incision is excellent, being particularly useful for Ramstedt's operation and for right or transverse colectomy. The surgeon may divide either or both rectus muscles. A transverse epigastric incision is also useful if the abdomen is broad, and it may be curved (upward convexity) to allow greater access to the upper abdomen.

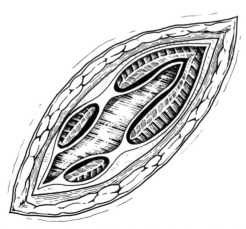

Fig 9.—Division of the rectus and oblique abdominal muscles along the length of the incision, in an outward direction for a short distance.

Lumbar sympathectomy can be accomplished via a transverse muscle-cutting incision that runs forward from the tip of the 12th rib to the lateral border of the rectus sheath with the patient tilted 30° to the opposite side. Muscle layers are divided down to but not including the peritoneum. Dissection then proceeds extraperitoneally, crossing the surface of the psoas muscle to the anterolateral aspect of the vertebrae. The ureter can also be approached via this incision and is found in a more anterior plane.

A slightly more oblique, open-curved, muscle-cutting incision may be made in either iliac fossa. This incision starts just above the anterior-superior iliac spine and all the tissues are divided in the line of the fibers of the external oblique muscle and aponeurosis. On the right it is known as the Rutherford-Morrison incision, which gives good access to a difficult inflamed appendix. A sigmoid colectomy can be performed via a similar incision on the left side, but access to the rectum is less satisfactory than if a vertical incision is used.

PFANNENSTIEL INCISION

This incision is frequently employed by gynecologists for access to the pelvic organs and is used in most cesarean sections. It is also employed in open retropubic prostatectomy since it gives excellent access to the retropubic space.

The skin incision is usually about 12 cm (5 inches) long, centered above the symphysis pubis and curved along the interspinous skin crease. The incision is deepened through the superficial fascia to expose both anterior rectus sheaths, which are divided along the whole length of the incision. Artery forceps (clamps) are placed on the upper and lower edges of each rectus sheath, and the sheath is then dissected widely, both above and below, from the underlying rectus muscles. The sheath is separated in an upward direction almost to the umbilicus and downward as far as the pubis. The rectus muscles are then separated in the midline and retracted laterally, and the peritoneum is opened vertically in the midline, commencing in the upper end of the wound, with care taken caudally not to injure the bladder. In the extraperitoneal approach to the prostate, blunt gauze dissection is carried out extraperitoneally to expose the bladder and prostate.

The great advantage of the Pfannenstiel incision is that it leaves an almost invisible scar which, in any case, is hidden by the pubic hair. The exposure is limited and the incision should only be used when the surgeon is certain that only pelvic intervention is necessary.

The laparotomy incision, whether upper midline, upper paramedian, or upper oblique, can be extended into either the right or the left chest, thus converting the pleural and peritoneal cavities into one common space. This gives excellent access on the right side for major hepatic surgery and on the left side for total gastrectomy or resection of the esophagogastric junction.

The patient is placed in the "corkscrew" position. The abdomen is tilted to about 45° by means of sandbags and the thorax is twisted into the full lateral position. This gives maximal access to both the abdominal and thoracic parts of the exposure.

The abdomen is opened through whichever upper abdominal incision the surgeon prefers and preliminary exploration of the abdomen is carried out to assess operability and to determine whether or not the thoracic part of the exposure is necessary. If it is decided to proceed to the full exposure, the abdominal incision is then continued along the line of the eighth interspace, which is identified as the space immediately distal to the inferior pole of the scapula. It is useful to infiltrate the line of the incision with 1:200,000 adrenalin solution.

The thoracic incision is carried down through subcutaneous fat and latissimus dorsi, serratus anterior, and external oblique muscles. The intercostal muscles of the eighth space are divided. It is helpful to use the diathermy needle throughout, in what is otherwise a rather vascular approach. The pleural cavity is opened and the lung allowed to collapse. The incision is continued across the costal margin and the cartilage is divided with a solid scalpel. Resection of a short segment of the costal cartilage allows easier subsequent closure of the chest wall. A self-retaining chest retractor is inserted and slowly opened to produce wide retraction of the intercostal space, so that it is not usually necessary to resect a rib. The diaphragm is divided radially after ligating branches of the phrenic vessels along the line of the incision.

DISRUPTION OF THE ABDOMINAL WALL

The choice of a particular abdominal incision, the choice of closure technique and the choice of suture material are largely colored by the safety of the wound healing which is to be achieved. At worst, failure results in total breakdown of the abdominal incision—"the burst abdomen"—or, less dangerous to the patient but still a troublesome complication, initial healing of the wound but subsequent development of an incisional hernia.

Before describing the technique of abdominal wound closure, we must discuss these two complications, with particular reference to their etiology.

BURST ABDOMEN

Disruption of the abdominal incision may be partial, wherein either the skin or the peritoneal layer remains intact but there is rapid development of a massive full-length incisional hernia, or complete, wherein all layers of the abdominal incision tear apart with or without protrusion of the abdominal contents (evisceration).

Incidence

The published incidence of burst abdomen varies between 0% and 3%. These days, most surgeons would regard the latter figure as extremely high, and a fair estimate for all cases would be less than 1%. The published reports require critical assessment. Some publications consider all laparotomies, including those performed through McBurney incisions. Reitamo and Moller,[5] for example, report a 10-year survey of laparotomies in Helsinki. Of 8,226 laparotomies, there were 49 burst abdomens (0.6%) but these included gridiron appendectomies, and if these are excluded, the incidence rises to 0.9%. Although dehiscence and herniation of McBurney's incisions may occur, they are most unusual. Some studies include only elective surgery and exclude emergencies and reopened abdominal wounds. Retrospective studies are less likely to be as accurate as prospective trials since one can never be sure that reviews of patient records will reveal every case of wound disruption. A patient who dies with a laparotomy wound kept together by the skin sutures but with gut exposed in its depths may not reach the hospital statistics.

Etiology

The abdominal wound may break down either completely or partially because of one or more of the following reasons:

1. *The knot may break or undo.* This is a technical error which is seen from time to time, although it should be avoidable by immaculate technique.

2. *The suture may rupture,* either because it is too weak for the tension placed on it or because it is rapidly destroyed in the tissues before adequate wound healing has taken place. This factor should be avoidable if suture material of the correct size and type is selected.

3. *The sutures may cut through the tissues.* This may occur either because they are placed too close to the wound edge or because of excessive weakening of the tissues from such factors as jaundice, uremia, protein depletion, or, most important, infection.

Wound breakdown is more likely to occur if the tension placed on the healing wound is increased by abdominal distention or by postoperative coughing or straining.

Although in some instances a single cause can be implicated, more often the cause of wound failure is multifactorial. Indeed, the clinical study of wound healing is complicated by the fact that it is unusual for a single cause to exist in isolation and it may be difficult to determine which of a number of factors has played the important part in wound breakdown. One can envision the not uncommon situation of a patient undergoing a laparotomy who is suffering from advanced abdominal malignant disease. He may be jaundiced, anemic, and protein depleted. After the operation he may develop an ileus with severe abdominal distention, and he may also have a postoperative cough from pulmonary collapse; in addition, he may be on cytotoxic treatment. On top of this, we must consider what part the choice of the incision, the type of suture material, the technique of closure and the experience of the surgeon may play.[6] It should be noted, also, that in any large series there will be a number of cases of wound disruption or herniation for which no obvious cause can be found.

Studies of large clinical series and, more importantly, the publication in recent years of results from prospective controlled trials have provided considerable information of a factual nature on the importance of various suggested etiologic factors.

Age and Sex

Burst abdomen is more common in patients over the age of 60 and in the male sex. Tweedie and Long,[7] in a study of 113 burst abdomens, noted a 2.6:1 male-female ratio of burst abdomen. However, on the general surgical service alone, the ratio increased to 6.7:1. Penninckx and colleagues[8] found a significant difference between males and females (.36% and 1.4%) in a study of 117 burst abdomens from Leuven, Belgium, while Lythgoe,[9] in 89 examples of complete disruption in Manchester, found a 3.7:1 male-female ratio. The majority occurred in patients in the sixth and seventh decades of life. Efron[10] found a male-female ratio of 2.2:1 in his study of 128 patients with burst abdomen at St. George's Hospital, London.

POOR TISSUE HEALING

It is an everyday observation that wound healing is rarely a problem in the heathy young patient undergoing a routine elective operation. Problems are likely to be met when the patient is obese or emaciated, elderly, infected, jaundiced, diabetic, anemic, alcoholic, protein depleted, vitamin C deficient, or suffering from any disease condition being treated with prolonged steroids. Two or more of these factors often coexist.

Vitamin C

Vitamin C is essential for collagen synthesis. In man, the vitamin C body pool of 2–3 gm is depleted in 90–120 days, to produce scurvy. Clinical scurvy is now uncommon, but less severe degrees of vitamin C deficiency may be found in patients with severe dysphagia, patients with peptic ulcer (who usually avoid eating fresh fruit and vegetables), and in dietary fadists. Man shares the dubious honor with the guinea pig of being unable to synthesize this vitamin, relying entirely on exogenous sources.

McGinn and Hamilton[11] showed that there is a fall in the level of vitamin C in the blood of patients following operation, which returns to normal in about 7 days. However, patients who received a blood transfusion during the operation have a persistently low vitamin C blood level. The leukocytes are responsible for both storage and transportation of ascorbic acid. Hemorrhage depletes this reserve and it is not replaced by stored blood, since the leukocyte ascorbic acid falls to a deficiency level after a week of bank storage. These authors suggest that this phenomenon may account for the increased incidence of abdominal wound dehiscence and anastomotic leakage that has been noted in patients undergoing emergency surgery for bleeding peptic ulcer.

Uremia

There is good laboratory evidence that uremia inhibits wound healing. Nayman et al.[12] found that laparotomy breakdown occurred in uremic dogs and could be prevented by renal dialysis. In our laboratory, Colin, Elliot, and Ellis[13] demonstrated in uremic rats a significant diminution in the bursting strength of laparotomy wounds and anastomoses of small bowel. We also demonstrated marked inhibition of fibroblast growth in culture containing uremic serum. Unfortunately, only a few clinical observations have been published on wound healing in uremic patients, but Androulakakis[14] noted that 7 of 12 patients with acute postoperative uremia following renal surgery suffered complete wound dehiscence, and Moffat and colleagues[15] reported five instances of wound dehiscence in 19 patients operated on while undergoing long-term peritoneal dialysis.

Jaundice

Bayer and Ellis[16] demonstrated that obstructive jaundice in the rat decreases the strength of abdominal wound healing and delays fibroplasia and angiogenesis. A recent important study from the Edinburgh Royal Infirmary by Armstrong and colleagues[17] compared wound healing in 373 patients undergoing operation for obstructive jaundice and 760 anicteric patients undergoing cholecystectomy. Reduced wound healing, manifested by a higher frequency of wound dehiscence (3.2% vs. 0.5%) and incisional hernia (10.3% vs 1.8%), was seen in the jaundiced patients. A raised plasma bilirubin level was not of independent significance in these cases, but reduced wound healing was associated with a low hematocrit, low plasma albumin level, a history of pancreatitis, a malignant obstructing lesion, and postoperative wound and/or abdominal sepsis. Interestingly, however, we have shown[18] that the addition of bilirubin to fibroblasts grown in culture media causes morphological changes in the fibroblasts and impairs the growth of cells. The addition of jaundiced human sera to the culture media also causes similar changes.

Other Factors

Because of the multifactorial situation in seriously ill patients in the majority of examples of burst abdomen, it is not surprising that a number of other individual factors are suggestive rather than definitely proved. For example, White and colleagues[19] found that almost half their cases of burst abdomen were in patients with malignant disease. Trapnell[20] noted a 9% incidence of burst abdomen in cases of pancreatitis submitted to abdominal exploration, a much higher incidence than would be expected. Pitkin[21] compared 300 obese women with 300 women of normal build undergoing abdominal hysterectomy. The only three wound disruptions occurred in the obese patients, although this did not reach statistical significance. Alexander and Prudden[22] found a low level of plasma protein (<3 gm) in 31 of 58 patients with burst abdomen, compared with 9% of normal controls.

Increased Abdominal Pressure

Increased intra-abdominal pressure, in conjunction with poor tissue healing and faulty surgical technique, may well precipitate wound dehiscence. Postoperative vomiting, hiccup, coughing, and distention may impose serious stress on the freshly sutured abdominal wound sufficient to produce dehiscence.

Combinations of Factors

Many authors have implicated a group of factors in producing wound break down. Thus, Greenburg and colleagues[23] identified the elderly male patient who is malnourished, has undergone alimentary tract surgery, and develops a severe postoperative chest infection as the person at highest risk of developing a burst abdomen. Alexander and Prudden[22] identified chest complications, postoperative distention, hematoma, and wound infection. Baggish and Lee[24] implicated chest infection, distention, and steroid therapy, but found no association with obesity, wound hematoma or infection, or diabetes in their gynecologic patients. Guiney and colleagues[25] implicated cough, distention, vomiting, and wound sepsis, as did Hampton.[26] In a series of 326 patients undergoing layered closure of laparotomy wounds, reviewed by Heddle and Ellis,[27] there were nine burst abdomens and 14 incisional hernias. We identified jaundice reaching statistical significance as an etiologic factor, but the wound failure rate was also higher in patients with postoperative wound infection, chest complications, postoperative ileus, and obesity, although none of these alone reached statistical significance.

TECHNICAL FACTORS IN BURST ABDOMEN

We must now consider the part played by purely technical factors in the etiology of wound dehiscence: the surgeon's choice of incision, choice of suture material, and technique of wound closure.

Until recently, much that was written on these topics was based on clinical impressions. In recent years, the conclusions drawn from these impressions have been greatly modified by the results of carefully planned prospective clinical trials. Indeed, on the surgical unit at Westminster Hospital, we have been involved in such trials continuously for the past decade.

THE INCISION

Until recently, many surgeons considered that midline incisions, particularly in the upper abdomen, were more likely to disrupt than paramedian or oblique and transverse incisions. This impression failed to take into consideration the fact that midline incisions are often employed to gain rapid access to the abdomen in desperate emergencies due to hemorrhage, trauma, or sepsis. The other, more complicated, incisions are more often used in elective procedures but are certainly not free from the risk of disruption. It is true, however, that the incidence of dehiscence with the McBurney muscle-splitting incision is extremely low. Incisional hernias may follow this incision, especially in the presence of infection and when a tube drain has been brought out through the wound.

When the various incisions have been studied in prospective trials, no advantage or disadvantage has been identified for any of the major laparotomy incisions except for the lateral paramedian incision.

For example, Greenall and colleagues[28] carried out a randomized controlled trial in which 579 patients were allocated either to a midline or to a transverse/oblique incision. A mass closure technique was employed, using nylon, wire, or polyglycolic acid sutures. There were two burst abdomens, both through the midline incision, but the incidence was only 0.4%. Recently Ellis, Coleridge-Smith, and Joyce[29] carried out a prospective randomized trial on 209 patients undergoing major laparotomy. Patients who were considered suitable for a transverse incision were randomly assigned to this incision or to a paramedian incision. Those who were considered to require a vertical incision were randomly assigned to a median incision or a paramedian incision. All wounds were closed by the mass closure technique using nylon. There was a single burst abdomen, which occurred in a patient with a paramedian incision.

The Leeds group has claimed exceptionally good results with the use of the lateral paramedian incision. Thus, Donaldson and colleagues[30] report not a single instance of burst abdomen in 850 patients operated on through this incision. It should be noted that two important groups of patients were excluded from the Leeds series—patients undergoing emergency laparotomy for severe hemorrhage and patients who had already been given benefit of a previous laparotomy so that additional operation was performed through the same incision. The same group[2] randomly assigned 207 patients undergoing laparotomy to a midline, medial paramedian, or lateral paramedian incision; and there was a single burst abdomen, in the midline group.

In 1983 a prospective randomized trial was carried out at Westminster Hospital, London, and Scarborough Hospital in Yorkshire (Table 1). In all, 430 patients undergoing laparotomy

TABLE 1.—Incidence of Wound Failure in Midline versus Lateral Paramedian Incisions

| | STUDY GROUP | | |
INCISION	Westminster	Scarborough	TOTAL
Midline			
No.	116	105	221
Bursts	0	0	0
IH	10*	10*	20†
Median age (range)	60 (18–89)	66 (16–89)	. . .
Wide paramedian			
No.	108	101	209
Bursts	1	1	2
IH	1*	1*	2†
Median age (range)	57 (13–98)	67 (19–86)	. . .

*$P < .02$ (χ^2).
†$P < .005$ (χ^2).
IH, incisional hernia.

were randomly assigned to midline incisions (22) or lateral paramedian incisions (209). Follow-up is now available for 1 year. There have been two burst abdomens, one at each hospital, and both in patients having a lateral paramedian incision. There have been 22 incisional hernias, 20 in patients having the midline and only 2 in patients having the lateral paramedian incisions ($P < .005$). The numbers at each hospital are broken down in Table 1. Despite the different geographic areas and different surgeons, the results are remarkably similar.

Thus the lateral paramedian cuts the incisional hernia rate from approximately 10% to 1% of major laparotomies.

Technique of Wound Closure

Many surgeons believe that an important factor in the closure of the laparotomy incision is meticulous suture of the peritoneal layer, and indeed, this has been stressed for many generations in the standard textbooks on surgery. However, it is known from many laboratory and clinical observations that peritoneal defects heal with extraordinary rapidity.[31] It is also a common observation that it may be very difficult to close the peritoneum, particularly in obese patients or if the operative conditions are not ideal, and yet these wounds may heal without any further problem. Moreover, surgical heretics have for many years carried out laparotomy closure without bothering to suture the peritoneal layer and have claimed no problems arising therefrom. The question is one of some importance. If suture of the peritoneal layer makes no difference in abdominal wound healing, then an unnecessary and occasionally difficult surgical step can be avoided. If, however, there should be a higher incidence of wound failure if the peritoneum is not sutured, the procedure must be retained. In the laboratory, Karipineni et al.[32] found no difference in the bursting strength of laparotomy incisions in dogs, whether or not the peritoneal layer had been sutured. We put this to the test of a controlled prospective randomized trial,[27] studying 162 patients in whom closure of midline and paramedian incisions was performed with catgut to the peritoneum and continuous nylon to the muscle sheath, compared with 164 patients in whom the peritoneal suture line was omitted. There were four instances of total dehiscence in the two-layer closure group (2.5%) compared with five in the one-layer closure group in which peritoneum was left open (3%). The difference was not statistically significant.

We are at present engaged in a prospective trial of closure of the wide paramedian incision with and without suture of the peritoneal layer. The reason for this trial is that the initiators of this incision[30] advocate peritoneal closure. To date we have performed 61 closures with and 66 without peritoneal suture, without a single example of burst abdomen in either group.

Mass Closure

One of the most significant advances in reducing the incidence of burst abdomen has undoubtedly been the introduction of the mass closure technique, in contrast to the meticulous layer-by-layer closure of the abdominal wall so often advocated. Jones et al.[33] in 1941 first popularized mass closure when they reported a burst abdomen rate of 11% in laparotomies closed in two layers with catgut and of 7% in laparotomies closed with catgut for the peritoneum and interrupted steel wire for the rectus sheath. In contrast, in 81 consecutive laparotomies closed with interrupted mass far and near sutures of steel wire, incorporating all layers of the abdominal wall apart from the skin, they had but a single burst abdomen. The far and near suture, in fact, was first used in 1900 by Smead, so that the technique of mass closure using the far and near suture is often referred to as the Smead-Jones technique.

Dudley[34] and Jenkins[35] have proposed theoretical arguments supporting the value of mass closure of the abdominal wound with nonabsorbable sutures and incorporating wide bites of tissue on either side of the incision line, a minimum of 1 cm from the wound edge. Clinical reports give strong support to theory. Goligher,[36] for example, reported only one instance of complete dehiscence in 108 elective laparotomies using interrupted wire sutures for all coats. Kirk[37] reported no disruptions in 186 laparotomies closed with mass continuous nylon, as did Martyak and Curtis[38] in 280 midline laparotomies and Leaper et al.[39] in 120 cases using wire. Jenkins[35] reported the excellent results of only one dehiscence in 1,505 closures using mass nylon suture.

Because of the excellence of these reports, we switched over to the mass closure technique in 1977. We employ No. 2 double nylon continuous suture to close the full thickness of the abdominal incision apart from skin, which is sutured separately with interrupted fine nylon. Bites are taken at least 1 cm from the edge of the wound and are placed close together, a maximum of 1 cm apart. Although we have not carried out a controlled trial comparing mass closure with layered closure, a study of our serial results is of some interest. From 1975 to 1977, 341 layered closures were performed, with 13 complete dehiscences (3.8%). From 1977 to 1980 the mass closure technique was used in 788 patients, with six burst abdomens, an incidence of 0.8% (Table 2).[46]

TABLE 2.—INCIDENCE OF WOUND HERNIATION RELATED TO SOME
SUGGESTED CAUSAL FACTORS*

FACTOR	ALL PATIENTS (N = 1,129)	PATIENTS WHO DEVELOPED HERNIAS (N = 84)	χ TEST
Patients:			
Mean age (yr)	46.1	58.2	$P < .001$
Men	510	62	$P < .0001$
Obesity	200	30	$P < .0001$
Taking steroids	20	1	NS
Jaundiced	45	3	NS
Incision:			
Midline	544	48	
Paramedian	558	35	} NS
Transverse	27	1	
Length > 18 cm†	155/419	31/36	$P < .001$
Suture:			
Mass (nylon)	684	49	NS
Mass (PGA)	104	12	$P < .05$
Two layer (catgut/nylon)	177	9	} NS
One layer (nylon)	164	14	
Surgeon:			
Consultant	424	18	} $P < .005$
Senior registrar	471	47	
Registrar	207	19	NS
Operation:			
Local antiseptic	867	63	NS
Drain	548	44	NS
Bowel surgery	378	43	$P < .01$
Malignancy	258	13	NS
Emergency	184	14	NS
Postoperative complications:			
Chest infection	195	32	$P < .0001$
Abdominal distention	148	24	$P < .0005$
Wound infection	179	41	$P < .00001$

*From Bucknall et al.[40] Reproduced by permission. Numbers in table refer to number of patients.
†Measuring commenced in 1978.

CHOICE OF SUTURE MATERIAL

Although for decades catgut was used extensively for closing major laparotomy wounds, a number of important controlled studies have demonstrated the high incidence of burst abdomen when this suture material is employed. Goligher et al.[41] reported a study of 319 patients undergoing elective paramedian laparotomies who were randomly assigned to catgut layered closure, catgut closure with tension sutures, and mass closure with interrupted wire sutures. There was a 10% incidence of burst abdomen in the first compared with just under a 1% incidence in the other two groups. Tagart[42] found a 3.4% incidence of burst abdomen when catgut was used for closure, compared with a 0.9% incidence when nylon was used. Leaper et al.[43] reported a

6.5% incidence of burst abdomen following two-layer closure with continuous catgut, and the incidence was just as high following mass closure with interrupted catgut.

Most surgeons, greatly impressed by published results such as these, have now switched to nonabsorbable sutures in abdominal wall closure. Wire gives excellent results but is difficult to use, and most now employ monofilament nylon.

Synthetic long-chain carbohydrate absorbable sutures have been introduced in recent years. The first of these was polyglycolic acid (PGA, Dexon). However, this material is known to lose about 80% of its strength within 2 weeks, whereas abdominal wall fascia requires approximately 120 days to regain its strength. In the randomized study by Bucknall and Ellis,[44] of 104 wounds closed with Dexon by the mass technique there was one burst abdomen and 12 incisional hernias (12.5% failure), compared with one burst abdomen and four hernias (4.7% failure) in the nylon group ($P < .05$) (see Table 2). Leaper et al,[43] also reported an 0.8% incidence of burst abdomen and an 8% incidence of hernia following mass closure with interrupted Dexon, compared with a 0% burst abdomen rate and a 5% incisional hernia rate following mass closure with steel wire. More recently a more slowly absorbed carbohydrate, vicryl polyglactin, has been developed which takes about 10–11 weeks to undergo complete absorption. However, Wasiljew and Winchester[45] report three burst abdomens in 272 laparotomies closed with this material.

It has been claimed that an advantage of absorbable sutures is a reduction in the rate of persistent sinus formation. However, in our own trial we found an 11.5% incidence of wound sinus in the Dexon group compared with 9.5% incidence in the nylon group.[40] The difference correlated with findings in an electron microscopic study that demonstrated that infection delays complete absorption of the Dexon, allowing it to act as a persistent foreign body.[46]

The choice of suture materials in abdominal wound closure will be discussed more fully in a later section.

MORTALITY FROM BURST ABDOMEN

Complete dehiscence of the abdominal wound is associated with a serious mortality, as high as 30% in some series, although most reports give an operative mortality in the region of 10%. It is not the wound dehiscence itself that is so lethal but the fact that this complication occurs so often in otherwise generally ill patients. This point was emphasized by Guiney et al.,[25] who noted that in most cases, the burst abdomen was only one of a number of factors that contributed to the fatal outcome in their study of 232 patients with a 15% mortality.

It should also be noted that incisional hernia following burst abdomen is not uncommon. For example, it occurred in no less than one third of patients in the series reported by Guiney and et al.

INCISIONAL HERNIA

Incisional hernias vary from a small insignificant bulge in the wound, revealed only on careful examination when the patient coughs, lifts the legs upward while in the lying position, or sits up, and may not even be noticed by the patient. At the other extreme, the rupture may be very large, unsightly, and uncomfortable. If the neck is narrow, there is the risk of strangulation, although this is unusual. Rarely, a large thin-walled hernia may become ulcerated, with protrusion of omentum or even the development of an intestinal fistula.

INCIDENCE

Many surgeons state that incisional herniation is a rarity. In some instances this may be due to excellence of the surgical technique. Goligher and colleagues[41] reported not a single incisional hernia in 108 laparotomies following mass closure with interrupted wire sutures, even though there was one burst abdomen in this group. Donaldson and colleagues,[30] using the lateral paramedian incision, reported only one incisional hernia in 231 selected laparotomies. However, we believe that in the majority of circumstances, the reported rarity of incisional herniation is due to the fact that patients are not followed up sufficiently and not examined carefully. Our definition of a hernia is any bulge at all in the wound when the patient is examined in the lying position and made to lift the legs upward, to sit up, and to cough. In a study of 1,129 major laparotomy wounds followed up for 12 months after operation[40] we detected a 7.4% incidence of incisional hernias. Others have reported similar findings; for example, Pollock[47] found a 10% herniation rate at 6 months in 961 patients, Johnson et al.[48] found a 13% incidence in 213 laparotomies followed up for 6 months, and Irvin et al.[49] found a 4.7% incidence at 6 months in 200 consecutive laparotomies.

Most investigators follow up their patients for 6 or at the most 12 months following laparotomy. We recently reported on 363 patients whose wounds had soundly healed at 1 year but whom we reviewed again between 2½ and 5½ years later.[50] No less than 21 of these patients (5.8%) were found on their follow-up examination to have developed incisional hernias. Six were unaware of the presence of the hernia and none was inconvenienced by it or requested surgical repair. Interestingly, none of the causal factors (which we will discuss later) was found to be associated with the development of these late hernias. It is difficult to explain how mature collagen can stretch to form an incisional hernia more than a year after sound healing has occurred. However, Harding et al.[51] from Cardiff, Wales, have also reported late development of incisional hernia in their investigation carried out 3 and 5 years after laparotomy. Akman,[52] in a study of 500 incisional hernias requiring surgery, noted that just over half were present within 6 months of the original operation. Three quarters had developed within 2 years of operation, and 97% were present within 5 years of the initial laparotomy.

ETIOLOGY

Our study of more than 1,000 consecutive laparotomies in which there were 19 complete dehiscences and 84 incisional hernias has enabled us to make careful observations on etiologic factors (see Table 2). Herniation was commoner at a statistically significant level in old patients, male patients, the obese, patients undergoing large bowel surgery, and patients with incisions longer than 18 cm. There was no significant correlation with the type of incision used (although this was before our study of the wide paramedian incision). Interestingly, there was no difference in incidence between wounds closed by consultants and registrars, although the incidence was higher following closure by senior registrars. The most significant factors were postoperative complications—chest infection, abdominal distention, and most important, wound sepsis. Forty-eight percent of the 179 patients in whom a wound infection developed also had an incisional hernia.

Our series included 104 patients whose laparotomies were closed with polyglycolic acid (Dexon), and in this group there were 11.5% wound herniations—a significantly higher percentage than in those closed by nylon.

In our trial comparing transverse, conventional paramedian, and midline incisions[29] there was no significant difference in herniation rates (Table 3).

TABLE 3.—INCIDENCE (%) OF WOUND HERNIATION BY INCISION TYPE

WOUND	CONVENTIONAL PARAMEDIAN	MIDLINE	TRANSVERSE
Intact	71	30	43
Hernia	15*	9*	7*
Total	86	39	50

*Not significant by χ^2 test.

The prospective study by Pollock[47] of 98 incisional hernias in 961 patients gave results similar to our own: the most important factors were chest complications, male sex, age over 65, and wound infection.

CHOICE OF SUTURE MATERIAL

The choice of suture material is frequently motivated by an emotional rather than a scientific thought process. This is due mainly to a lack of knowledge by the surgeon of the physical and biologic properties of individual suture materials, and of the relevance of these properties to the clinical situation, where rates of healing and tissue response vary considerably. Certainly surgical technique is more important than the suture material, but a detailed knowledge of the material selected will lead to a more scientific approach to the problem of abdominal closure and, one hopes, to consistent and reproducible results.

CLASSIFICATION OF SUTURE MATERIALS

A wide variety of sutures are available with a broad range of physical and chemical configuration. Measurement of the in vivo degradation time provides a general classification. Sutures that undergo degradation in tissues, rapidly losing their strength within 60 days, are considered "absorbable." Sutures that maintain strength longer than 60 days are termed "nonabsorbable."

The absorbable materials are catgut and collagen, which occur naturally, and the synthetic polyglycolic acid polyglactin (Vicryl), and polydioxanone (PDS). Nonabsorbable sutures by definition are not absorbed, but some, especially those of biologic origin—for example, silk, cotton, and linen—lose strength rapidly after the second month and by 6 months have either disintegrated or are so weak as to have little power in reinforcing the tissues.[53, 54] Until 1930 these materials, together with catgut, were the only ones in common use. Steel wire was introduced in 1932 and synthetic nonabsorbable materials during and after World War II, starting with nylon in 1941. Modern chemistry had developed fibers derived from polyester (Dacron), polyamide (nylon) and polypropylene (Prolene). With these materials there is only minimal loss of tensile strength or change in mass following implantation.

The classification can be broadened by reference to the structure of suture materials. Some are monofilament and others multifilament, where the multifilament is either braided or twisted to form a suture. Finally, the surface characteristics can be altered by the application of coatings, some of which will reduce the capillarity of the suture material, while others will alter its coefficient of friction by reducing the drag factor and hence ease the passage of sutures through tissue, as well as facilitate knotting.

SUTURE SELECTION

The purpose of a suture is to hold the wound in apposition until such time as the healing process is sufficiently far advanced as to make its continued presence in the tissues unnecessary. The surgeon will always be faced with a large selection of suture materials and will have to make a decision as to which is the best material for a particular surgical procedure. The holding together of a wound for the initial postoperative period is entirely dependent on the suture. However, as healing progresses, the contribution made by the suture gradually decreases until finally it is redundant, since the support function has been taken over by the healing wound. Fascial tissue can take as long as 9 months to regain even 75% of its original tensile strength.[55] Therefore a nonabsorbable or an absorbable material with prolonged tensile strength retention is advisable for abdominal wall closure. If healing is long-delayed or incomplete, as in an infected wound,[56] support by sutures will be required for an even longer period.

It is advisable to keep the volume of the suture to a minimum, since all suture materials are foreign bodies. The smallest size of suture material that will hold the tissues in apposition without breaking should be used, and the correct knot should be tied to maintain security. The ideal knot for synthetic materials is a double throw followed by a single throw followed by another double throw. Additional throws on the knot increase the foreign body volume, and many extrusions and suture sinuses result from large knots.

Tissue reaction is an important aspect of suture selection. An exudative foreign body reaction and local tissue autolysis provides a protein-rich material which may facilitate bacterial growth and movement. The least reactive suture should always be chosen.

All suture materials show a difference between the knot pull strength and the straight pull strength. When a knot is placed on a suture material, the strength of the knot can be 10%–40% weaker than the unknotted strand, depending on the material. When a suture fails it always breaks at the knot, unless some damage has been inflicted on the material. The commonest cause of this damage is iatrogenic: the knot breaks because of rough handling, defective surgical instruments, or inadvertent crushing. Monofilament polypropylene is especially prone to damage by instruments.

Sterilization of suture materials also alters their characteristics. Most suture materials are sterilized by gamma irradiation from a cobalt 60 source or by ethylene oxide gas. Sterilization reduces the tensile strength by approximately 10%. Repeated sterilization can lead to sutures that have a low tensile strength and may account for subsequent failure in use.

Another important physical characteristic of suture material is its extensibility. This is the amount of "give" or stretch in a material, or elongation before the breaking point is reached. Many materials will return to their original length following extension short of breaking, while others will remain elongated; nylon is the prime example of the latter. Some materials can elongate as much as 30% before breaking and hence are useful where postoperative edema is expected to occur, and the "give" in the suture prevents cross-hatching on the underlying tissue.

A SUTURE FOR THE SPECIFIC TASK OF ABDOMINAL WALL CLOSURE

Moynihan[57] in 1920 proposed the requirements for an ideal suture material: it should be free from infection, be nonirritant to tissue, achieve its purpose, and, if appropriate, disappear when its work is finished. As we have seen, this ideal does not exist, and we must therefore choose the best material available for the given task of closing the abdominal wall.

Wound dehiscence, herniation, and sinus formation have been shown to be closely related to suture choice as well as to infection.[58] Catgut, for example, was rejected as the suture of choice following alarmingly high burst abdomen rates,[41] which are to be expected because of its poor tensile strength profile. We have therefore searched experimentally and clinically for the best available alternative.

Keill et al.[59] reported a 72.3% wound infection rate before bursting, compared to 3.4% for normal wounds, and in our series infection was the most significant factor associated with wound failure.[60] We should therefore look for the ideal suture available for a potentially infected abdominal closure (see Table 2).[60]

To reduce the rate of sinus formation and of wound failure, it is important to consider whether some suture materials are more likely to potentiate infection than others. Alexander et al.[61] implanted different types of suture materials into subcutaneous pouches of rabbits, inoculated with staphylococcal solution, and measured the diameter of the resulting abscesses. They concluded that the nonabsorbable monofilaments (monofilament nylon, wire, polyethylene) encourage less infection than catgut or multifilamentous materials. This technique, however, leaves much to be desired, and therefore James and MacLeod[62] introduced a technique of "infectivity" testing of sutures by measurement of the number of bacteria a suture length picked up from a bacterial solution. We have improved this technique and applied it to the sutures commonly used for abdominal wall closure.[58, 60]

Our results showed that braided black silk will pick up three times more bacteria from culture than the same length of monofilament nylon. Braided nylon results were very similar to those of silk, thus supporting recent studies showing that braided nylon is accompanied by infection just as often as silk.[63] Nylon is known to have low absorptive powers, yet braided nylon has a high capillarity due to its multifilamentous nature,[64] thus indicating that the ability to pick up organisms is related to the physical braided nature rather than the simple absorptive capability of the suture material. The number of bacteria picked up by PGA (which is braided) was intermediate between the numbers picked up by silk and monofilament nylon, possibly because the breakdown products of PGA may affect bacterial growth.[65]

The increased reaction and abscess formation in relation to infected sutures seen on light microscopy with silk, multifilament nylon, and PGA may again be attributed in part to the braided nature of the material and the persistence of bacteria in the interstices of the braid. The significance of the tissue reaction is not only that it produces delay in healing and a predisposition to infection but that it leads to a phenomenon known as "cutting out," in which, because of the reaction around the suture, the tissue strength is not great enough to maintain the suture in position. When a wound becomes infected the tissue reaction is known to be greater and hence the risk of the suture "cutting out" is higher. Because the strength of the wound is entirely dependent on the suture during the lag phase and a variable part of the healing phase, the importance of choosing a suture that will not "cut out" can be readily appreciated.

Van Winkle and Salthouse[66] postulated that multifilament sutures provide a haven for bacteria which, after penetrating the interstices of the suture, are "safe" from granulocytes and macrophages too large to work their way between tightly packed strands. The scanning electron microscope provided the opportunity for us to look at this theory. Sutures were implanted into the back of rats previously infected by local injection of *Staphylococcus aureus*. Sutures were removed at 10-, 30- and 70-day intervals and examined under the electron microscope.

Bacteria were found in the interstices of all multifilamentous material. However, this was particularly marked with silk (Fig 10) and multifilament nylon (Fig 11). Monofilament nylon showed a minimal zone of reaction and a thin fibrous covering which appeared early on (Fig 12). The reaction was slightly more cellular with infected sutures, but a capsule had still

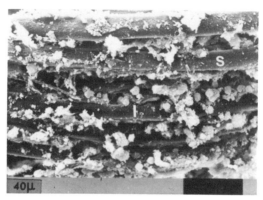

Fig 10.—Infected silk at 30 days. A marked polymorphonuclear leukocyte reaction *(I)* is seen between the strands *(S)* (reference scale, 40 μ).

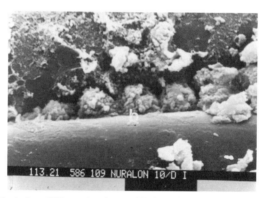

Fig 11.—Infected multifilament nylon at 10 days. Note cellular infiltration between strands. Leukocytes are seen with attached "grape-like" clusters of staphylococci *(b)* (reference scale, 10 μ).

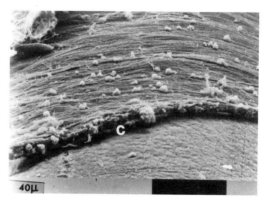

Fig 12.—Noninfected monofilament nylon at 30 days. A narrow band of fibrous tissue is forming a capsule *(c)* (reference scale, 40 μ).

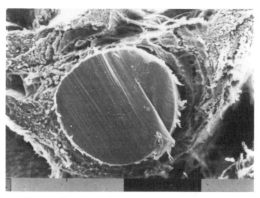

Fig 13.—Infected monofilament nylon at 30 days. There is a slightly increased cellular component, compared with noninfected suture, but still only a very narrow reaction zone. A fibrous capsule has developed (reference scale, 200 μ).

formed by 10 days (Fig 13). Multifilament nylon showed less reaction than silk when not infected (Figs 14 and 15). The strands were tightly bound at 70 days (Fig 16); however, the infected suture showed pus cells between the strands at 70 days (Fig 17). Silk showed a marked reaction even in the noninfected state (Fig 18). Giant cells appeared earlier in the noninfected suture (Fig 19), possibly due to the presence of a polymorphonuclear reaction, continuing in the infected suture to 70 days (Fig 20). PGA showed little cellular reaction in a noninfected state (Fig 21) until giant cells invaded and quickly appeared to absorb the suture, leaving a "ghost-like" capsule at 70 days (Fig 22). The giant cell invasion process was again slowed by the polymorphonuclear cell reaction to infection (Fig 23). There was less absorption, and suture strands were still present at 70 days (Fig

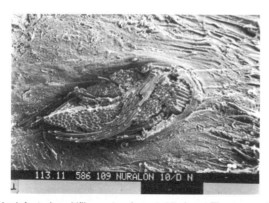

Fig 14.—Noninfected multifilament nylon at 10 days. The zone of response is slight. The suture strands remain tight, with little tendency for cellular infiltration (reference scale, 400 μ).

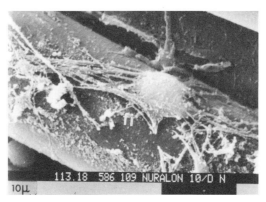

Fig 15.—Noninfected multifilament nylon at 10 days. Fibroblasts *(fi)* and occasional giant cells are seen in an otherwise "clean" suture (reference scale, 10 μ).

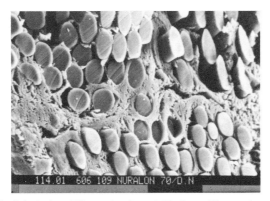

Fig 16.—Noninfected multifilament nylon at 70 days. Fibrous tissue ingrowth is seen around the outer strands. A well-defined fibrous capsule surrounds the whole structure (reference scale, 40 μ).

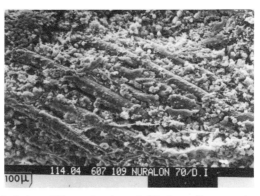

Fig 17.—Infected multifilament nylon at 70 days. Pus remains between the strands (reference scale, 100 μ).

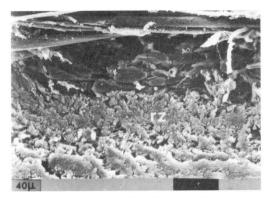

Fig 18.—Noninfected silk at 10 days. There is a prominent reaction zone *(rz)* even when not infected (reference scale, 100 μ).

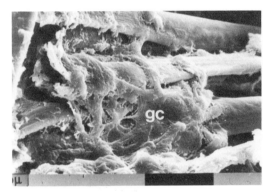

Fig 19.—Noninfected silk at 70 days. Filaments have been almost completely engulfed by giant cells *(gc)* (reference scale, 20 μ).

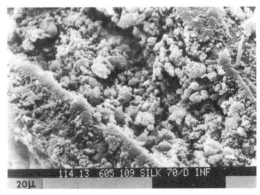

Fig 20.—Infected silk at 70 days. There is a marked infective reaction (reference scale, 20 μ).

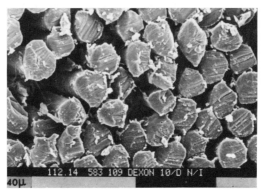

Fig 21.—Noninfected PGA (Dexon) at 10 days. There is no absorption at this time. Strands are still tightly packed, with very little cellular reaction (reference scale, 40 μ).

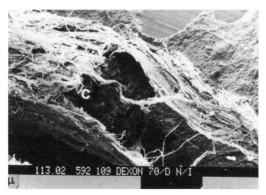

Fig 22.—Noninfected PGA (Dexon) at 70 days. There is 80% absorption, with a hollow appearance of the capsule *(c)* (reference scale, 200 μ).

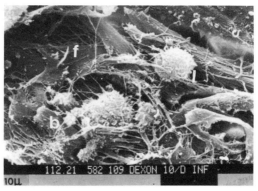

Fig 23.—Infected PGA (Dexon) at 10 days. The zone of reaction is greater than in Figure 13, with a marked cellular infiltration of the strands. Polymorphonuclear cells *(l)* are seen with attached strands of fibrin *(f)* and bacteria *(b)* (reference scale, 10 μ).

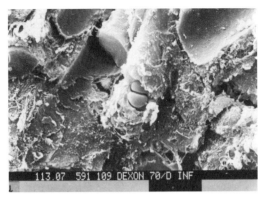

Fig 24.—Infected PGA (Dexon) at 70 days. Only 50% of suture is absorbed. The cellular component is greater than in the noninfected PGA (see Fig 14) (reference scale, 10 μ).

24). These strands were therefore acting as foreign bodies without any strength.

The reaction around monofilament nylon was therefore minimal; there was nowhere for the bacteria to hide, unless, of course, the suture was knotted.

We know that less bacteria are required to produce a wound infection when a suture is present.[67] Therefore, perhaps one other theoretical disadvantage of sutures that retain bacteria is that polymorphonuclear leukocytes, which are important in the early phases of healing, are drawn away from the wound to combat the infection in the suture, with subsequent slowing of wound healing.

When the tensile strength of a wound is measured with the sutures in situ, a characteristic curve is obtained, as described by Howes and Harvey in 1929.[68] During the first 3–4 days there is a decline in strength—as much as 50% of the initial strength may be lost. This is termed the lag phase. It is followed by a period of increasing tensile strength, termed the healing phase. During the lag phase and a considerable part of the healing phase, the strength of the wound is entirely dependent on the sutures. It is therefore fundamental that a suture material should retain adequate strength for the purpose for which it is used. In abdominal closure, where it takes many months for fascia to heal, durability of sutures is of particular importance. In our studies, using an Ingstrom tensiometer to test the strength of sutures, prepared as for the electron microscopic investigations, we found that nylon in both monofilament and braided forms retained its strength during the complete test period of over 70 days. Silk sutures, normally regarded as being nonabsorbable, in fact lost up to 83% of their original strength after 70 days. This confirms the work of Postlethwaite,[69] who found that naturally occurring fibers compare unfavorably with synthetic ones in terms of durability. PGA sutures rapidly lost strength after implantation, and by 30 days only 4% of the original strength remained. Infection slowed its absorption. However, as it takes well over 70 days for an abdominal wound to heal, the results for PGA were disturbing.

The initial experimental and clinical work with PGA was highly encouraging. The material has tensile strength of the order of multifilamentous polyester (Mersilene).[70, 71] It handles like silk and has a very low tissue reactivity, calling forth mainly a giant cell response prior to complete disappearance from the tissues at 60–90 days.[71,72] However, tensile strength loss does not parallel absorbability, and in PGA the tensile strength loss is complete at 30 days.

The nearest to the ideal suture of those tested was monofilament nylon. Its strength should be sufficient to hold abdominal wall fasciae together, even if healing is delayed by infection. It does not disappear (in the literal sense of the word) when its work is finished but it does become walled off quickly in a fibrous capsule, even in the presence of infection. It is inert and nonirritating to tissue and least likely to act as a nidus for bacterial infection.

One problem with monofilament nylon is that it has a "memory" and tends to uncoil and take its original form; therefore, a multiple throw knot is needed for security. Because of this problem, surgeons have recently been using the monofilament polypropylene (Prolene), a suture with similar properties to nylon but without such a good memory. However, Postlethwaite[73] reported that Prolene has a 4% fragmentation rate, and 2.6% of Prolene sutures left in situ for 5 years exhibit bone and cartilage formation in the rim of fibrous tissue.

The Role of Sutures in Clinical Practice

Wound dehiscence occurs if sutures are unable to hold the wound edges together until the wound has acquired sufficient strength of its own through the healing process.

The use of absorbable material involves an increased risk of wound dehiscence. We have already reviewed the unacceptably high rate of burst abdomens when catgut alone was used. Insufficient strength of nonabsorbable suture material is seldom the cause of wound dehiscence, but inadequate knot tying technique may cause this complication.[74] The causes of sutures cutting through supporting tissue are not fully understood, but certainly one important factor is weakening of the supporting tissue by lysis of collagen.[75] Increased lysis of collagen is caused, for example, by inflammatory reaction in the tissue elicited by infection or by suture material, or both. The work of Howes[76] has helped to eliminate this problem. He suggested that large bites should be taken. Jenkins[35] applied simple arithmetic to this need, and from 1957 to 1973, using two layers of continuous monofilament nylon, he closed 1,500 major laparotomies and had only one burst abdomen. He penetrated the tissues with needle and sutures at 1.1- to 1.3-cm intervals and used deep bites. By measuring the unused length of the continuous nylon suture and the total length of the wound (and subtracting the length of unused nylon from the total suture length), he found that the ratio of suture length used to wound length closed varied from 3.5 to 5.3 for the suture length to 1 for the wound length. Each stitch therefore required 4 to 6 cm of material, confirming the fact that bites 1 to 1.5 cm deep had been taken, as indicated. In seven patients not in the series, three with burst abdomens and four with incisional hernias, he found that the ratio of suture length to wound length was less than 2:1, indicating that the sutures had been inserted too near the cut edges.

In spite of the cogent theoretical[34] and practical[77, 78] arguments in favor of mass closure, Ellis[79] reported that many surgeons still closed laparotomies in layers, and rates of burst abdomen of 3% or more were not uncommon.

When the Smead-Jones interrupted mass closure technique or the continuous deep bite technique with monofilament steel,[39, 78] monofilament nylon,[36–38, 40, 44, 80] or polypropylene [81] is used, wound dehiscence occurs in less than 1% of laparotomies.

Dudley[80] states that early disruption occurs because sutures cut through shortly after operation, and late hernia may result if the suture material used disappears before sufficient collagen has been laid down to restore intrinsic strength. The first can be avoided if sufficiently large bites are taken, the second if nonabsorbable material is used.

PGA sutures had been used in the same way and have been shown to be equally effective,[39, 82] but these patients had only a short follow-up.

In a clinical trial in which we compared monofilament nylon with PGA for the mass closure of abdominal wounds[44] and followed up the patients for more than a year, there was a significantly higher wound failure rate with PGA. In particular, there was an 11.5% hernia rate with PGA, compared with only 3.8% hernia rate with nylon ($P < .05$). Also, the expected advantage of the absorbable PGA suture, in terms of zero sinus formation rate, was not seen (11.5% with PGA, 9.5% with nylon), presumably due to infection, which delayed the complete absorption of the suture. In most circumstances the strength of PGA suture is sufficient to hold the fascia together. However, with delayed healing due to infection or with raised intra-abdominal pressure due to postoperative chest infection or abdominal distention, the strength of the wound without suture support may be insufficient, leading to the formation of an incisional hernia. The persistence of absorbable suture material after its strength has gone means that it continues to act as a foreign body without providing support in any way. Add to this the inertness of the modern nonabsorbable synthetic sutures, and there is little theoretical reason for recommending absorbable suture for closing the abdominal wall.

We have illustrated that the choice of suture material has a significant bearing on the success of abdominal wall repair. There is no question that if one selects a large enough suture, even though the suture is absorbable, satisfactory closure can be obtained. All one has to do is be sure that the absorbable suture does not dissolve in less time than is needed for adequate tensile strength to develop. The question that cannot be answered, however, is why take the chance? To see how close one can come to failure without actually doing so has never made as much sense as seeing how far one can stay from failure. Closure of the abdominal wall is an exercise in maintaining and developing tensile strength of scar tissue. Why not give the patient the greatest possible insurance against loss of tensile strength in the suture before wound healing has produced a safe scar?

SINUS FORMATION

Early attempts to exploit the greater sustained tensile strength of nonabsorbable sutures were thwarted by the frequency with which stitch sinuses occurred when natural nonabsorbable sutures (for example, silk) were used. A local abscess or chronic granulomatous reaction occurs around the suture, resulting in a discharging sinus, which clears up only when the suture is removed or extruded. The frequency of this complication is directly related to the degree of contamination. Cutler and Dunphy[83] in 1941 found sinus rates of 2.3% in clean wounds closed with silk and 11% in contaminated wounds, but this figure rose to 80% in infected wounds. However, monofilament stainless steel wire rarely produces sinuses in clean wounds[84, 85] unless the suture breaks.[86]

If a monofilamentous material, for example nylon, is used in infected wounds, the incidence of sinus formation is between 6% and 12%.[85, 87] The incidence in our study, in which monofilament nylon was used, was 9.4%.

The theoretical advantage of an absorbable suture in this respect is obvious. Leaper et al.[39] in 1977 reported a zero incidence of sinuses when using PGA, and Bentley et al.[82] in 1978 found that only 1% of their 814 abdominal wounds closed with PGA developed sinuses. We have found that the incidence of sinus formation was much higher, 11.5%, when PGA was used. The

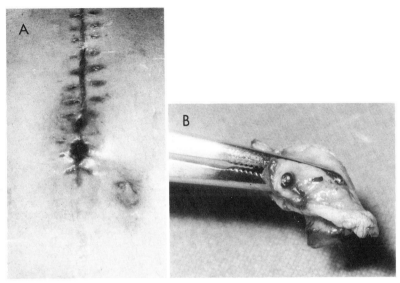

Fig 25.—**A,** abdominal wound sinus caused by a knotted suture. **B,** excised suture knot.

reason for this high incidence is not clear, but perhaps represents the effects of infection on the PGA suture which prevent its total fragmentation and absorption.

Knots always provide space in which bacteria can become enmeshed, and the knot is the commonest site of wound sinus formation in clinical practice (Fig 25). A method of sealing knots would be a real advance.

Wound infection, however, remains the most significant factor associated with sinus formation, and efforts must continue to eliminate this serious complication.

TECHNIQUES OF CLOSURE

The ideal method of closure of the abdominal wound remains to be discovered. It should be technically easy and rapid to perform; entirely free from the complications of dehiscence of the abdominal wound, incisional hernia, and persistent sinuses; comfortable to the patient; and leave an all but invisible scar.

Closure of the McBurney right iliac fossa muscle split incision and the Pfannenstiel incision most closely approaches these ideals. With major laparotomy incisions, work over the past decades has greatly reduced the risk of burst abdomen, but incisional hernia formation and persistent sinuses are still far from uncommon.

McBurney Incision Closure

Because this is a muscle-splitting incision, the divided oblique muscles snap together again once the muscle relaxant has worn off, and in fact the wound will heal safely if only the skin is sutured. Most surgeons, however, including ourselves, feel more reassured if a simple closure technique is employed.

A quick and effective technique is to pick up the edges of the divided peritoneum with artery forceps (clamps) and close the peritoneum with a simple catgut purse string suture, having first brought down the omentum beneath the wound to prevent the possibility of small bowel becoming adherent to the scar. There is no need to close the internal oblique and transversus muscle, but one, or at the most two, interrupted sutures of No. 1 catgut appose the divided external oblique aponeurosis. No sutures are placed in the subcutaneous fat, and the skin edges are drawn together with fine interrupted nylon sutures or closed with clips or staples.

Pfannenstiel Incision

Conventionally, the peritoneum is closed with catgut and the rectus sheath with Dexon or nylon. Probably the peritoneal closure could be omitted, and this assertion is based on studies in which we left the peritoneal layer open in a series of midline and paramedian incisions without deleterious effects.[27] However, we have not seen reports of controlled trials in which this layer has been omitted in the Pfannenstiel incision.

Midline and Paramedian Incisions

We have discussed the controversies concerning layered closure versus mass closure and the extensive studies that have been made of the various types of suture material. Based on the studies we have described and discussed, we advocate the mass closure technique using nylon.

It is now fully realized, both from clinical studies and from animal experiments, that healing of the incision takes place by the formation of a dense fibrous scar that unites the apposing faces of the laparotomy wound. The purpose of the sutures is to splint the wound edges while this dense fibrous scar deposits and matures. Wide bites must be taken at a minimum depth of 1 cm from the edge of the wound and placed at intervals of less than 1 cm from one to the next. The suture length employed should measure at least four times the wound length, in order to ensure an adequate reserve of suture length in the wound when this is placed on tension, as may occur during abdominal distention.[35]

Where possible, omentum is drawn down to cover the abdom-

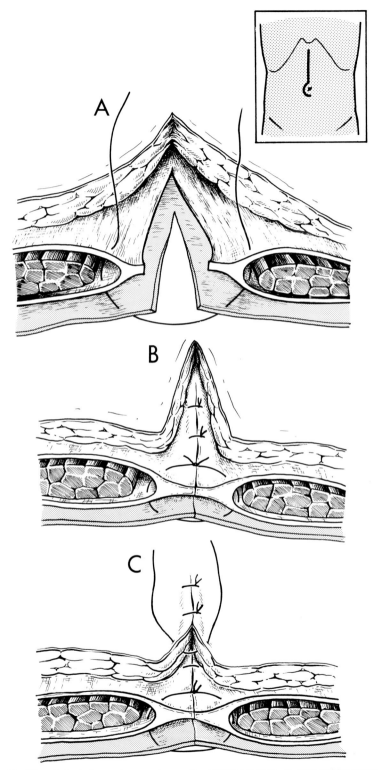

Fig 26.—A, technique of mass closure for midline wounds. **B,** optional interrupted mass suture. **C,** simple skin closure with interrupted nylon.

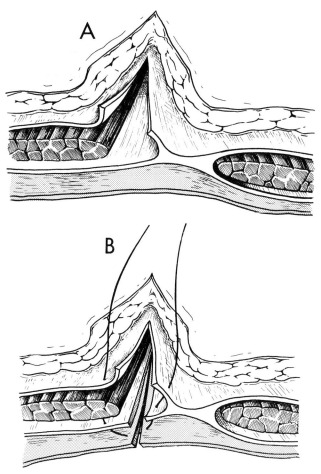

Fig 27.—A, conventional paramedian incision. **B,** mass closure of a paramedian incision.

inal viscera before closure is commenced in order to prevent adhesions between small bowel and the deep layer of the laparotomy incision. We use a hand-held large Moynihan five-eighths needle in order to take wide bites of the full thickness of the abdominal wall and employ No. 1 nylon. For the midline incision, all layers of the abdominal wall apart from skin and subcutaneous fat are included in the suture, the skin then being closed with interrupted nylon (Fig 26). A similar technique is used for the paramedian incision, picking up the anterior and posterior rectus sheath (Fig 27). The transrectus incision incorporates the medial portion of the rectus muscle in the suture loops. Transverse oblique and Kocher incisions can also be safely closed with this mass nylon technique. If the peritoneum cannot be included in the suture, this is of no consequence, as was demonstrated in our controlled trial study.[27]

Some surgeons employ interrupted nylon sutures, either placed simply or by the far and near Smead-Jones technique. To date, we have discovered no evidence showing that interrupted sutures have any advantage over the continuous technique, which is certainly a more rapid method. We are at present engaged in a controlled randomized trial comparing continuous nylon with interrupted nylon sutures in cases where a previous laparotomy incision is re-employed at a second laparotomy. This trial has been in progress for less than a year. Forty-two reopening laparotomies have been performed to date, 16 closed by the interrupted and 26 by the continuous technique. So far there have been three incisional hernias, two in the interrupted and one in the continuous group. We anticipate that at least another year will be necessary to recruit sufficient patients and another year for follow-up before any firm conclusion can be reached.

Donaldson et al.,[30] in describing the wide paramedian incision, advocated closure of the posterior rectus sheath together with peritoneum using catgut, and separate closure, with nylon, of the anterior rectus sheath. In our study of this incision, we have used that technique, but since the beginning of 1984 we have been engaged in a trial to determine whether or not closure of the peritoneal layer is necessary. So far (January 1985), in 66 cases of laparotomy through the wide paramedian incision *without* peritoneal closure, no incisional hernias have occurred.

THORACO-ABDOMINAL INCISION

The diaphragm is closed in two layers using continuous thread or Dexon. An underwater tube drain is placed in the pleural cavity through a separate stab incision in the ninth intercostal space and held in place with a purse string suture. The thoracic incision is then closed by suturing the chest wall muscles in layers using catgut or Dexon. There is no need to pass sutures circumferentially around the ribs, a technique that may give rise to a good deal of chest pain. The abdominal part of the incision is then closed by the mass suture technique using nylon and the skin is closed with interrupted fine nylon sutures.

We have not described the use of tension sutures in closure of the abdominal wall because we never employ this technique in primary closures of the abdominal wound. It is painful, gives rise to an ugly scar, and there is no evidence in any controlled trial of any value of these sutures in either preventing burst abdomen or incisional hernia if the mass closure technique is employed. The only use for tension sutures is in closure of a burst abdominal incision in those cases where the wound edges are infected and necrotic.

REFERENCES

1. Ellis H.: Midline abdominal incisions. *Br. J. Obstet. Gynaecol.* 91:1, 1984.
2. Guillou P.J., Hall T.J., et al.: Vertical abdominal incisions: A choice? *Br. J. Surg.* 67:395, 1980.
3. McBurney C.: The incision made in the abdominal wall in cases of appendicitis: With a description of a new method of operating. *Ann. Surg.* 20:38, 1894.
4. Kocher T.: *Textbook of Operative Surgery,* ed. 2. London, Black, 1903.
5. Reitamo J., Moller C.: Abdominal wall dehiscence. *Acta Chir. Scand.* 138:170, 1972.
6. Ellis H.: Management of the wound, in Schwartz S., Ellis H. (eds.): *Maingot's Abdominal Operations,* ed. 8. New York, Appleton-Century-Crofts, 1984.
7. Tweedie F.J., Long R.C.: Abdominal wound disruption. *Surg. Gynecol. Obstet.* 99:41, 1954.
8. Penninckx F.M., Poelmans S.V., et al.: Abdominal wall dehiscence in gastroenterological surgery. *Ann. Surg.* 189:345, 1979.
9. Lythgoe J.P.: Burst abdomen. *Postgrad. Med. J.* 36:388, 1960.
10. Efron G.: Abdominal wound disruption. *Lancet* 1:1287, 1965.
11. McGinn F.P., Hamilton J.C.: Ascorbic acid levels in stored blood in patients undergoing surgery after blood transfusion. *Br. J. Surg.* 63:505, 1976.
12. Nayman J., McDermott F.T., Gurr G.W.: Wound dehiscence in acute renal failure. *Med. J. Aust.* 1:799, 1969.
13. Colin J.F., Elliot P., Ellis H.: The effect of uraemia upon healing: An experimental study. *Br. J. Surg.* 66:793, 1979.
14. Androulakakis P.A.: Uraemia and wound healing. *Br. J. Surg.* 67:380, 1980.
15. Moffat F.L., Deitel M., Thompson D.A.: Abdominal surgery in patients undergoing long-term peritoneal dialysis. *Surgery* 92:598, 1982.
16. Bayer I., Ellis H.: Jaundice and wound healing: An experimental study. *Br. J. Surg.* 63:392, 1976.
17. Armstrong C.P., Dixon J.M., et al.: Wound healing in obstructive jaundice. *Br. J. Surg.* 71:267, 1984.
18. Taube M., Elliot P., Ellis H.: Jaundice and wound healing: A tissue culture study. *Br. J. Exp. Pathol.* 62:227, 1981.
19. White H., Cook J., Ward M.: Abdominal wound dehiscence: A ten year survey from a district general hospital. *Ann. R. Coll. Surg. Engl.* 59:337, 1977.
20. Trapnell J.: Management of the complications of acute pancreatitis: *Ann. R. Coll. Surg. Engl.* 49:361, 1971.
21. Pitkin R.M.: Abdominal hysterectomy in obese women. *Surg. Gynecol. Obstet.* 143:532, 1976.
22. Alexander H.C., Prudden J.F.: The causes of abdominal wound disruption. *Surg. Gynecol. Obstet.* 122:1223, 1966.
23. Greenburg A.G., Saik R.P., et al.: Wound dehiscence. *Arch. Surg.* 114:143, 1979.
24. Baggish M.S., Lee W.K.: Abdominal wound disruption. *Obstet. Gynecol.* 46:530, 1975.
25. Guiney E.J., Morris P.J., Donaldson G.A.: Wound dehiscence: A continuing problem in abdominal surgery. *Arch. Surg.* 92:47, 1966.
26. Hampton J.R.: The burst abdomen. *Br. Med. J.* 2:1032, 1963.
27. Heddle R., Ellis H.: Does the peritoneum need to be closed at laparotomy? *Br. J. Surg.* 64:733, 1977.
28. Greenall M.J., Evans M., et al.: Midline or transverse laparotomy? A random controlled trial. *Br. J. Surg.* 67:188, 1980.
29. Ellis H., Coleridge-Smith P.D., Joyce A.D.: Abdominal incisions: Vertical or transverse? *Postgrad. Med. J.* 60:407, 1984.
30. Donaldson D.R., Hegarty J.H., et al.: The lateral paramedian incision: Experience with 850 cases. *Br. J. Surg.* 69:630, 1982.

31. Ellis H.: The aetiology of post-operative abdominal adhesions. *Br. J. Surg.* 50:10, 1962.
32. Karipineni R.C., Wilk P.J., Danese C.A.: The role of the peritoneum in the healing of abdominal incisions. *Surg. Gynecol. Obstet.* 142:729, 1976.
33. Jones T.E., Newell E.T., Brubaker R.E.: The use of alloy steel wire in the closure of abdominal wounds. *Surg. Gynecol. Obstet.* 72:1056, 1941.
34. Dudley H.A.F.: Layered and mass closure of the abdominal wall. *Br. J. Surg.* 57:664, 1970.
35. Jenkins T.P.N.: The burst abdominal wound: A mechanical approach. *Br. J. Surg.* 63:873, 1976.
36. Goligher J.C.: Visceral and parietal sutures in abdominal surgery. *Am. J. Surg.* 131:130, 1976.
37. Kirk R.M.: Effect of method of opening and closing the abdomen on incidence of wound bursting. *Lancet* 2:352, 1972.
38. Martyak S.N., Curtis L.E.: Abdominal incision and closure: A systems approach. *Am. J. Surg.* 131:476, 1976.
39. Leaper D.J., Pollock A.V., Evans M.: Abdominal wound closure: A trial of nylon, polyglycolic acid and steel sutures. *Br. J. Surg.* 64:603, 1977.
40. Bucknall T.E., Cox P.J., Ellis H.: Burst abdomen and incisional hernia: A prospective study of 1129 major laparotomies. *Br. Med. J.* 284:931, 1982.
41. Goligher J.C., Irvin T.T., et al.: A controlled clinical trial of three methods of closure of laparotomy wounds. *Br. Med. J.* 62:828, 1975.
42. Tagart R.E.B.: The suturing of abdominal incisions: A comparison of monofilament nylon and catgut. *Br. Med. J.* 54:952, 1967.
43. Leaper D.J., Rolenberg I.L., et al.: The influence of suture materials on abdominal wall healing assessed by controlled clinical trials. *Eur. Surg. Res.* 8(suppl. 1):75, 1976.
44. Bucknall T.E., Ellis H.: Abdominal wound closure: A comparison of monofilament nylon and polyglycolic acid. *Surgery* 89:672, 1981.
45. Wasiljew B.K., Winchester D.P.: Experience with continuous absorbable suture in the closure of abdominal incisions. *Surg. Gynecol. Obstet.* 154:378, 1982.
46. Bucknall T.E.: Factors influencing wound complications: A clinical and experimental study. *Ann. R. Coll. Surg. Engl.* 65:71, 1983.
47. Pollock A.V.: Laparotomy. *J. R. Soc. Med.* 74:480, 1981.
48. Johnson C.D., Bernhardt L.W., Bentley P.G.: Incisional hernia after mass closure of abdominal incisions with Dexon and Prolene. *Br. J. Surg.* 69:55, 1982.
49. Irvin T.T., Stoddard C.J., et al.: Abdominal wound healing: A prospective clinical study. *Br. Med. J.* 2:351, 1977.
50. Ellis H., Gajraj H., George C.D.: Incisional hernias: When do they occur? *Br. J. Surg.* 70:290, 1983.
51. Harding K.G., Mudge M., et al.: Late development of incisional hernia: An unrecognised problem. *Br. Med. J.* 286:519, 1983.
52. Akman P.C.: A study of five hundred incisional hernias. *J. Int. Coll. Surg.* 37:125, 1962.
53. Douglas D.M.: Tensile strength of sutures: Less when implanted in living tissue. *Lancet* 2:499, 1949.
54. Moloney G.E.: The effect of human tissues on the tensile strength of implanted nylon sutures. *Br. J. Surg.* 48:528, 1961.
55. Douglas D.M.: The healing of aponeurotic incisions. *Br. J. Surg.* 40:79, 1952.
56. Bucknall T.E.: The effect of local infection upon wound healing: An experimental study. *Br. J. Surg.* 67:851, 1980.
57. Moynihan B.G.A.: The ritual of a surgical operation. *Br. J. Surg.* 8:27, 1920.
58. Bucknall T.E.: Abdominal wound closure: Choice of suture. *J. R. Soc. Med.* 74:580, 1981.
59. Keill R.H., Keitzer W.F., et al.: Abdominal wound dehiscence. *Arch. Surg.* 106:573, 1973.

60. Bucknall T.E., Teare L., Ellis H.: The choice of a suture to close abdominal fascia. *Eur. Surg. Res.* 15:59, 1983.
61. Alexander J.W., Kaplan J.Z., Altemeier W.A.: Role of suture materials in the development of wound infection. *Ann. Surg.* 165:192, 1967.
62. James R.C., Macleod C.J.: Induction of staphylococcal infections in mice with small inocula introduced on sutures. *Br. J. Exp. Pathol.* 42:266, 1961.
63. McGeechan D., Hunt D., et al.: An experimental study of the relationship between synergistic wound sepsis and suture materials. *Br. J. Surg.* 67:636, 1980.
64. Blomstedt B., Osterberg B.: Fluid absorption and capillarity of suture materials. *Acta Chir. Scand.* 143:67, 1977.
65. Thiede A.: Controlled experimental histological and microbiological studies on the inhibition of infection by polyglycolic acid. *Chirurg* 51:35, 1980.
66. Van Winkle W., Salthouse T.N.: Biological response to sutures and principles of suture selection. Scientific exhibit, American College of Surgeons Clinical Congress, San Francisco, 1975.
67. Flek S.D., Conen P.E.: The incidence of *S. pyogenes* in man: A study of the problems of wound infection. *Br. J. Exp. Pathol.* 42:266, 1957.
68. Howes E.L., Harvey S.C.: The strength of the healing wound in relation to the holding strength of the catgut suture. *N. Engl. J. Med.* 200:1285, 1929.
69. Postlethwaite R.W.: Long term comparative study of non-absorbable sutures. *Ann. Surg.* 171:892, 1970.
70. Herrmann J.B., Kelly R.J., Higgins G.A.: Polyglycolic acid sutures. *Arch. Surg.* 100:486, 1970.
71. Katz A.R., Turner R.J.: Evaluation of tensile and absorption properties of polyglycolic acid sutures. *Surg. Gynecol. Obstet.* 131:701, 1970.
72. Postlethwaite R.W.: Polyglycolic acid surgical suture. *Arch. Surg.* 101:489, 1970.
73. Postlethwaite R.W.: Five year study of tissue reaction to synthetic sutures. *Ann. Surg.* 190:54, 1979.
74. Hawes E.L.: Strength studies of polyglycolic acid v. catgut sutures of the same size. *Surg. Gynecol. Obstet.* 137:15, 1973.
75. Holmlund D.E.W.: Suture technique and suture holding capacity: A model and a theoretical analysis. *Am. J. Surg.* 134:616, 1977.
76. Howes E.L.: The immediate strength of the sutured wound. *Surgery* 7:24, 1940.
77. Higgins G.A., Antkowiak J.G., Esterkyn S.H.: A clinical and laboratory study of abdominal wound closure and dehiscence. *Arch. Surg.* 98:421, 1969.
78. Irvin T.T., Stoddard C.J., et al.: Abdominal wound healing: A prospective clinical study. *Br. Med. J.* 2:351, 1977.
79. Ellis H.: Wound healing. *Ann. R. Coll. Surg. Engl.* 59:382, 1977.
80. Dudley H.A.F.: Laparotomy. *Br. J. Hosp. Med.* 14:577, 1975.
81. Herrmann R.E.: Abdominal wound closure using a new polypropylene monofilament suture. *Surg. Gynecol. Obstet.* 138:84, 1974.
82. Bentley P.G., Owen W.J., et al.: Wound closure with Dexon (PGA) mass suture. *Ann. R. Coll. Surg. Engl.* 60:125, 1978.
83. Cutler E.C., Dunphy J.E.: The use of silk in infected wounds. *N. Engl. J. Med.* 224:101, 1941.
84. McCullum G.T., Link R.F.: The effect of closure techniques on abdominal disruption. *Surg. Gynecol. Obstet.* 119:75, 1964.
85. Shouldice E.E., Glassow F., Black N.: A study of sinuses occurring after the use of silk only, wire only or a combination of the two. *Can. Med. Assoc. J.* 84:576, 1961.
86. Robinson J.R.: Closure of abdominal incision with continuous steel sutures. *Am. J. Surg.* 84:690, 1952.
87. Usher F.C., Allen J.E., et al.: Polypropylene monofilament: A new biologically inert suture for closing contaminated wounds. *JAMA* 179:780, 1962.

SELF-ASSESSMENT ANSWERS

1. *a,, c*
2. *a, b, c*
3. *True.* The sinus formation rate is 2% in clean wounds, 11% in contaminated wounds, and up to 80% in infected wounds when silk is used.
4. *c*
5. *b*
6. *False*
7. *True*
8. *b, d, e*
9. *a*
10. *a*